MIND, BODY AND SPIRIT
A Holistic Guide to Healthier Living

ELAINE DESTINY-BEY

ISBN: 978-1537432601

Contact author at:
Elaine Destiny-Bey
P. O. Box 36484
Las Vegas, Nevada 89133
elainedestinybey@gmail.com

Affirmations: Powerful, uplifting, manifesting words

Chakras: Learn about the 7 gateways to heaven

Meditation: How to meditate and balance your chakras

☥

DEDICATION

This book is dedicated to all spiritual beings spirit-man, spirit-woman and spirit-child.

Table of Contents

☥

Affirmations

AFFIRMATIONS are powerful, uplifting words, and manifesting words. These words change how we feel and how we view ourselves. We can uplift ourselves with positive words and change our subconscious minds. The more we speak something, the more we become what it is that we are speaking. Our words are powerful and we have the power to make change into our lives.

Here are some examples of affirmations. (Be creative and feel free to come up with your own).

1. I love and approve of myself.

2. I follow my intuition and my heart keep me grounded.

3. I make the right choices every time.

4. I draw from my inner strength and light.

5. I trust myself.

6. I trust my inner wisdom and intuition.

7. I breathe in positive energy and breathe out negative energy.

8. All situations have a divine purpose and work out for my highest good.

9. Wonderful things unfold before my own eyes.

10. I can see clearly.

11. I refuse to give up because I haven't tried all possible ways.

12. I know my wisdom guides me in the right decision.

☥

13. I trust myself to make the best decision for me.

14. I love without judgement.

15. I am a beautiful, vibrant, spiritual being full of light and energy.

16. I am in-tune with the universe.

17. I respect my body, mind and spirit.

18. I am able to receive love and give love because I am love.

19. I am in a divine state of mind.

20. I am a powerful force of electric light.

21. I have a sacred temple.

22. I speak sacred words.

23. I am a natural healer.

24. I will only eat live foods that will be nourishment for my body.

25. Divinity is my way of life.

26. Peace dwells in me.

27. I live by Maat.

28. I will not take part in any gossip.

29. I am on a high frequency.

30. Meditation is my medication.

31. My mind is the most powerful tool.

32. I use my time wisely.

33. I deserve all of the fortunes life has to offer.

34. I make connection with light spiritual beings.

☥

35. I have harmony in my life.

36. I always use my higher self for thinking.

37. I am one with the divine.

38. The universe provides for me.

39. I am open to unlimited possibilities.

40. I am the creator of my own destiny.

41. I am the best.

42. I am legendary.

"The purpose of all human life is to achieve a state of consciousness apart from bodily concerns."
~Kemetic Proverbs~

☥

What Are Chakras?

Chakras are the energy centers in our body, through which energy flows. Each one of us has 7 major chakras in our body. I like to call them spiritual centers. These energies flow rapidly, spinning in circular motion if they are in balance. Chakras stay balanced and open by spiritual practices. People who practice spiritual things daily are usually in alignment and balance with the universe.

Having a blocked chakra could affect you in so many different ways. You may feel tired, weak, low of energy, negative, emotional, stressed, sick, etc. That's why one should keep their chakras vibrating on a natural rhythm that keeps everything balanced. You can balance your chakras by meditating, praying, chanting, speaking words of affirmations, fasting, eating healthy foods, exercising, getting energy healing work done (reiki), and living in Maat.

"The conscious heart of a human is his or her own God."
~Kemetic Proverbs~

☥

The Seven Major "Spiritual Centers" Known As Chakras

Crown Chakra
"Spirituality"
Associated color is **Violet**
The crown spiritual center is the 7th chakra. This chakra deals with the higher self. It's the direct connection with the divine (God). This chakra is located right on top of your head. This is a very sensitive area for us because all divine guidance is received through this chakra. We can receive positive or negative energy through this center. Our life force energy flows down from the crown to the rest of the spiritual centers. If this chakra is balance you will have a deeper connection with your higher self.
Crystals: Amethyst, white topaz, clear quartz, white calcite

Third-Eye Chakra
"Awareness"
Associated color is **Indigo**

The third-eye spiritual center is the 6th chakra. The third-eye chakra usually deals with psychic abilities and intuition. This chakra is marked in between the middle of brows in the center of the forehead. This chakra is associated with the pineal gland. The pineal gland in ancient times was considered the spirit of man. Balancing this chakra with bring clairvoyance, psychic connection, spiritual communication, and development of intuition. Overall, you can see the known or the un-known with your third-eye.

Crystals: Amethyst, fluorite, azurite, celestite, lapis lazuli, benitoite, clear quartz

Throat Chakra
"Communication"
Associated color is **Blue**
The throat chakra spiritual center is the 5th chakra and this chakra deals mainly with expression/communication. The throat chakra brings forward creativity, speech, expression and communication. If one has any throat problems or they need help with verbal communication this is the chakra to balance and clear. By clearing and balancing you begin to think clearly, speak your truth, and connect with spirit.

☥

Crystals: Lapis lazuli, turquoise, blue lace agate, blue tourmaline, clear quartz

Heart Chakra
"Love"
Associated color is **Green**
The heart spiritual center is the 4th chakra. This chakra deals with love. The heart chakra brings balance, harmony, affection and love to one's life. The heart chakra is the balance point for all spiritual centers. This chakra can bring new loving relationships. Also, this chakra can help one to connect back to nature. If one wanted to heal a broken heart this is the chakra to work with.
Crystals: Rose quartz, emerald, malachite, green jade, pink sapphire, clear quartz

Solar Plexus
"Wisdom"
Associated color is **Yellow**

The solar plexus spiritual center is the 3rd chakra. This chakra deals with who you are. It is located at your core right above your navel. Balancing this chakra can help with your self-confidence, personality, and will power. Working with this chakra you will come into awareness of your personal life purpose.

Crystals: topaz, citrine, yellow zircon, amber, lemon quartz, clear quarts

Sacral Chakra
"Sexuality"
Associated color is **Orange**
The sacral spiritual center is the 2nd chakra. This chakra usually deals with feelings and is the center of all creativities, as well as connecting to all of your emotions, pleasures, and sexuality. If one needs help with accepting oneself or creating new ideas, this chakra is the chakra to work with.

Crystals: Amber, citrine, fire agate, orange carnelian, clear quartz

Root Chakra
"Grounded"
Associated color is **Red**

☥

The root spiritual center is the 1st chakra. This chakra deals with mainly things of the lower self. All physical activities and your strength comes from this chakra. Usually, this chakra deals with sexual activities and reproduction organs. While keeping you grounded, this center helps you connect back to earth. If you are having troubles with feeling safe and secure this is the chakra to work on.

Crystal: ruby, red jasper, blood stones, rose quartz, garnet

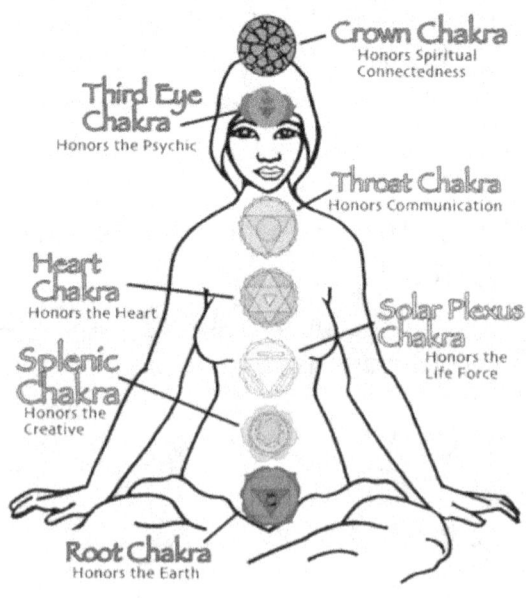

"As above, so below, we are created in the image of NETER (GOD)."
~Kemetic Proverbs~

☥

What is Meditation?

Meditation is an experience of relaxing the body, quieting the mind, and awakening your inner spirit.

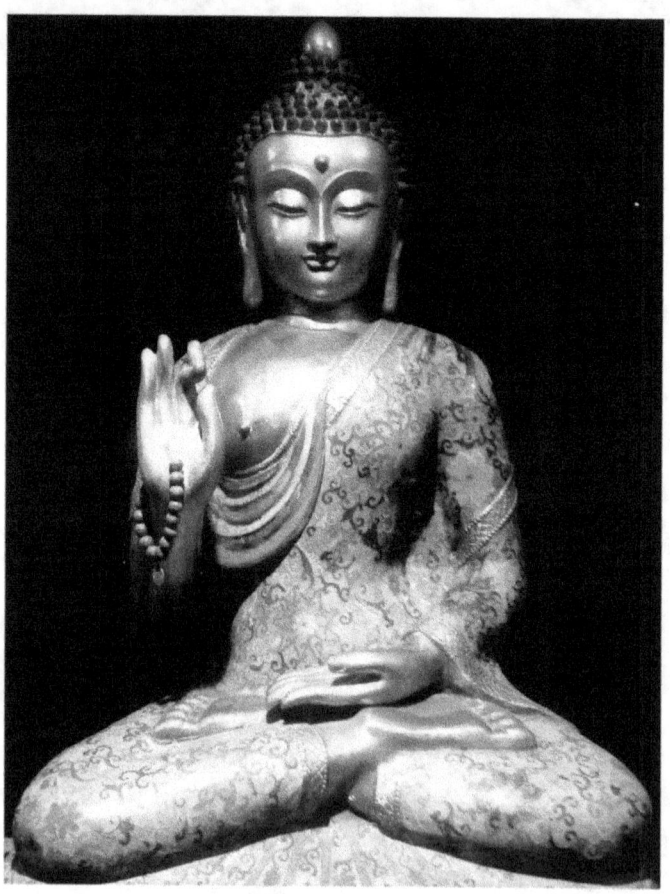

Benefits of Meditation

1. Helps to balance your chakras
2. Gives you a sense of purpose
3. Opens up your third-eye
4. Improves focus and alertness
5. Promotes better relations for the mind, body, and spirit
6. Increases your happiness and inner peace
7. Helps you focus on the present moment, promoting concentration
8. Helps reduce stress, depression, and anxiety
9. Builds self confidence
10. Promotes healing
11. Increases blood circulation
12. Helps with breathing
13. Relaxes nervous energy
14. Promotes awareness of self
15. Keeps you in harmony and Maat

☥

When Should You Meditate?

The best time for your meditations, or any spiritual practices, is the first thing in the morning or upon waking up. One should give thanks to the creator of their liking. Pray and then meditate. In my opinion, meditation is like medication. It's spiritual healing for the mind, body, and spirit. There is no perfect time to do meditation. However, the best time to do this is before the sunrise. This will help promote a positive day ahead. Overall, whenever you can meditate it beats not meditating at all. If you can do it in the morning, thumbs up. If you cannot do it in the morning then do it in the afternoon, evening or just before bedtime. Whatever time is perfect for you. All is well. Just use meditation to become conscious, and raise your vibrations. This technique and spiritual practices will help you see things clearly.

"Mediation technique is also the easiest to learn and has the most enjoyable rewards. One would absolutely enjoy this spiritual practice. This should become a part of one's daily lifestyle."
Buddha

☥

How to Meditate

One meditation is medication for the spirit raising up on vibrations, but one must know how to meditate.

1. **Space**
   Find your sacred space. This place could be your bedroom, living room or outside in nature. This place should be a place where there is quietness, and you can be comfortable. This place should be relaxing and free from distractions. You can sit in silence or add meditation music. Do what is best for you.

2. **Posture**
   Posture is everything when it comes to meditation. It is recommended to have your spine in an upright position with your head up. Sitting in a chair or sitting in Indian style helps connect the body with your mind. Also, it helps to activate your pineal gland. If your body is in balance, then your mind will fall in

place. So, sitting upright, letting the energy flow up and down your spine, activates each of the spiritual gateways (chakras).

3. **Eyes**

It's best during medication to close your eyes. This helps with relaxation and calmness, allowing you to drift off into a meditative state. Seeing with your eyes closed enables you to see with your mind. However, it's important to do what makes you comfortable.

4. **Thoughts**

Let your thoughts be clear and emotions be balanced. Do not over think it. Mediation is very easy to do if you relax and let go of the present. Just let your mind be free and focus on your breathing. Spirituality is the act of breathing. Concentrating on the breathing helps keep you from having

☥

random thoughts. The more you meditate the better you will become.

5. Time

Do not focus on time, just go within and let your spirit guide direct you. Try not to beat yourself up about doing 2-3 hours of meditation. Just do what you can. If it's 15 minutes, let that 15 minutes be your best 15 minutes. Every minute counts towards balancing your mind, body, and spirit. Just enjoy, meditation gets better over time.

6. Visualization

After, you have mastered the breathing part of meditation, you can begin to do some visualization. I find that visualizing yourself in nature connecting to the elements can be helpful for freeing your mind. Visualizing all the chakra colors penetrating each chakra in your body can help bring balance, and clear each chakra from blockage.

Envision them: the crown is violet, third-eye is indigo, throat is blue, heart is green, solar plexus is yellow, sacral is orange, and root is red.

7. **Healing**

Overall, meditation is healing for mind, body, and spirit. Promoting chakra balancing, raising ones vibration, having clear vision, and having a peace of mind all can be accomplished through meditation. Each one of us patiently seeks oneness with the divine, and meditation helps you get there. Make meditating a part of your lifestyle.

☥

"Everything is formed by habit, even praying."
~Kemetic Proverbs~

Breathing Techniques

Breathing before meditation helps you to relax, stay focus, and remain balanced. Also, breathing helps activate your pineal gland, release toxins and, stress, promotes circulation, and enhance intuition. Breathing techniques can be utilized every day to enhance ones energy.

Top Breathing Techniques

1. **Inhale/Exhale**
   Inhale through your nostrils, raising up your chest coming from diaphragm. On the count of 7. Hold a second on 7 than slowly release your breathe through your nostrils. Lowering your chest and feeling your body release tension.

2. **Fire Breaths**
   It is breathing in and out of your nostrils very rapidly. This helps to raise up your energy force (sekhem). One should gradually take their time and practice

☥

this technique. For beginners it could make them feel light headed.

3. Subtle Breathing

Subtle breathing is silent, relaxed, and naturally done. It is when the breathing is unrestrained, slowed down, and peacefully done. You just breathe and let nature take its course. The key to subtle breathing is to calm your mind, relax and let it rest in its natural state.

"Healing Crystals"

Crystals have been around for millions of years. Crystals carry high vibrations and energies just like humans. Some of the minerals that are in these crystals resides within us as well. These precious jewels can be utilized to help balance us out. Crystals promote healing for the mind, body and spirit.

Healers of all kinds have been utilizing crystals not for their beauty but for their spiritual and healing attributes. In my healing work I utilize crystals for healing, balancing the chakras, clearing the aura, protection from negative energy and so forth. You can meditate with them, astro travel with them, and bathe with them (spiritual bath) to reap some of the benefits. Just by having them on you or near you, one can benefit from their magnetic powers. The easiest way to inner-stand the powers of different crystals is to learn about them, their colors, and healing powers. Just see which ones draw you towards them.

There are thousands of different crystals on the planet. This list includes of a few I like to work with for balancing the Chakras.

☥

Amethyst

Provides a connection to the divine. Stimulates spirituality and contentment, reputes evil thought, great for meditation opening up that "Third Eye."

Rose Quartz

Often called, the "Love Stone." The fair and lovely Rose Quartz has a gentle pink essence; it is a stone of the heart, a stone of unconditional love. This stone stimulates the "Heart Chakra." If you would like to attract new love, romance, and intimacy this is the right crystal for you.

Moon Stone

Nick named the "Goddess Crystal." Helps with female problems such as menstrual, hormones, childbirth. Helps balance stability, stress and anxiety. Moonstone is a powerful tool enhancing psychic abilities, great for meditation.

Smoky Quartz

Is a Protection and Grounding crystal. It is also an excellent crystal for protection from negative energy, as it removes negativity and negative energy of any kind and transforms it to positive energy. Smoky Quartz is a "Root Chakra."

Bloodstone

Improves physical strength, enhances self-esteem and self-appreciation. Enhance creativity and intuition. Bloodstone provides aid in treating blood disorders and strengthens the immune system. This crystal enhances a person health and well-being.

Clear Quartz

Stimulating the Crown Chakra, Clear Quartz helps aid us with the source of spirituality, connecting us back to a higher plan of existence. This crystal could be utilized for protection. Clear Quartz brings balance, energy and harmony to one's life. This crystal balances all chakras.

☥

Lapis

One of the oldest spiritual stone known to mankind. This stone stimulates psychic abilities and inner vision. It represents universal peace. Lapis stone helps with spoken word, written word, and deep communication. This is a "Throat Chakra" stone.

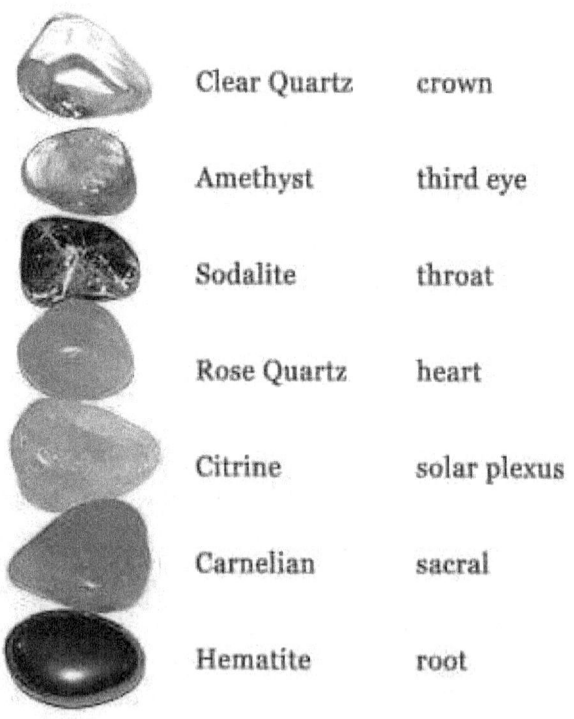

	Clear Quartz	crown
	Amethyst	third eye
	Sodalite	throat
	Rose Quartz	heart
	Citrine	solar plexus
	Carnelian	sacral
	Hematite	root

Recipe for Spiritual Bath

To clean your body from negative energy run a bath with sea salt, Himalayan pink salt or Epsom salt and say: "Salt and water purify me from negative energy and anything that does not serve my highest good. Let this water be healing, for my mind, body and spirit. Cleanse and hydrate every cell in my body." Ase' and so it is.

Ingredients:
6 drops of Lavender oil
6 drops of Frankincense oil
5 tablespoon of Epsom salt
1 white candle (white is for purity)
Add your favorite crystals to the water or around the tub
Add relaxing music

Pray and state your intentions while in the water. Water carries powerful vibrations. Make this time peaceful and relaxing. Meditate and listen to your inner-guide.

☥

"Sound Therapy"

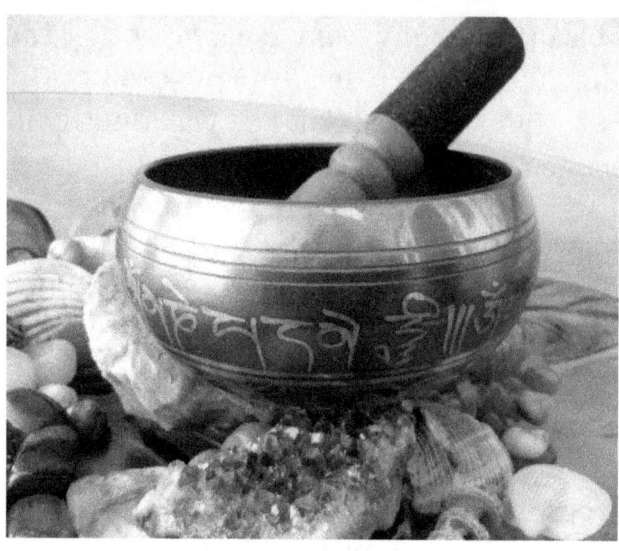

We utilize sound for healing. Sound carries different energy vibrations that promote different healing for the mind, body, and spirit. Since we as human spiritual beings are energy, sound helps to raise up that energy force. Sound therapy influences our emotions and physical behavior naturally. Instruments such as the drums have been used by indigenous people of Africa for spiritual rituals, ceremonies, and healing rituals for thousands of years and continue to be used this way by many cultures.

Sounds affect us each day, from bird sounds, water sounds, nature sounds, and musical instruments. Music sounds make us want to dance, snap our fingers, and jump up and down. They say music is for healing of the soul. You can hear a nice beat and instantly dance. Please, I encourage you to incorporate some form of sound therapy, such as singing bowls, drums, rattles, tuning forks, meditation sounds, or radio music for healing.

☥

Aerobic Exercise

Aerobic exercise is for the body. Also, known as physical exercise of low to very high intensity depending on which aerobic exercise one would like to do. Increase your oxygen level and promote more circulation by moving your body. The body was designed to move. Increase your energy level by incorporating physical activities (aerobic exercise) to your lifestyle. Physical movement is known to increase metabolism and longevity. Just moving your body more lowers your blood pressure, enhances oxygen flow, promotes circulation, maintains diabetes, cholesterol, weight, and keeps your bones strong. Better yet, physical activity releases stress, and toxins from the body.

To enhance your holistic lifestyle, physical activity 3x to 5x a week for 30 minutes a day is more than enough for healthy living. Whatever you would like to do whether it's jogging, swimming, cycling, yoga, tai chi, skating, jumping rope, dancing, or walking. Just move your body more, and start reaping the rewards.

Eat To Live

Eat to live is not just a catch phrase. Literally, the title speaks for itself. If you are not eating to live you are doing the very opposite of that and that, living to eat. Many of us have been trained to just eat because of taste, emotions, what is pleasing to the eyes, and social reason. That's bad because we do not pay attention to what we are actually eating. The foods we are eating are deteriorating our life. What foods are bad for our health? Fast foods, processed foods, canned foods, boxed foods, high in sugar foods, meat of all kinds, GMO foods, dairy, and most conventional fruits, and vegetables.

Fast food serves no nutritional value what so ever. It's high in fat, salt, cholesterol, sugar, corn syrup, and many more additives. Fast food is leading us to early death. Obesity is on the rise. Fast food is not good for human consumption. Please, say no to Mc' Donald's, Taco Bell, Jack-N-Box, KFC, etc. Do your research on more vegan/vegetarian, organic produce, and vegan restaurants, or just cook and prepare nutritional food at home.

☥

"Dangers of Meat"

Meat is very hard on the human digestion system, causing bloating for several days. Also, you are eating dead foods, which causes you to feel tired, and it brings down your vibrations and lowers your immune-system. On a spiritual note, if it has a mother do not eat it. The meat now has several chemicals in it that lead to cancers, heart disease, and immune-disorders. They use chemicals and substances like arsenic, food coloring, steroids, growth hormones, antibiotics, and the list goes on. Please, do your research on the dangers of meat and try to eliminate meat all together.

Whole foods is what one should be eating to live. Whole foods are our natural foods that give us life, energy, and nourishment for our bodies. Foods that absorb the sun and have been organically grown, such as fruits, and vegetables are what one should be eating for life. Alkalize your body by adopting a vegan/vegetarian diet.

What are the benefits of being a vegan/vegetarian:

- **Maintaining weight**
- **Better cholesterol levels**
- **Longer life**
- **Lower risk of cancers, obesity, and heart disease**
- **Alkalize your body**
- **Absorb minerals and vitamins**
- **Have a healthy digestion system**
- **Gain more energy**
- **Look younger**
- **Build up your immune system**
- **Less toxin absorption**
- **Natural detox**

Transition yourself to a healthier diet by choosing to **"Eat To Live!"**

☥

HERBAL MEDICINE

Genesis 1:29

Then God said, "I give you every seed bearing plant on the face of the whole earth and every tree that has fruit with seed in it. They will be yours for food."

Many people have lost the ancient ways of living, especially when it comes to healing. People have become accustomed to western medicine. No one is asking questions and doing the proper research when it comes to health related issues. Most people just go to the professional doctors who practice medicine. We do what we are told by the health care professionals. Does a man know by being told? The majority of the time we are taking some type of prescription medicine to treat our symptoms.

Many of these pharmaceutical drugs have many side effects, which can make things worse by treating one aliment but making another get worse. I realize there are not any cures in westernized medicine. The majority of these drugs stabilize the disease and over time this leads to cancers, tumors, and chronic illnesses due to medications. This is why I choose to do things using a more holistic approach. One way of doing this is taking herbs.

Herbs are any plants with leaves, seeds or flowers. They can be used for food, medicine, or fragrances. Herbs have been around for millions of years. Herbs are filled with many vitamins. They are nourishment for the body. Anyone could take them, and there are not any major side effects. Herbs are natural and they come from the Earth.

Western medicine is the newest form of medical practice. Western medicine has been around for about 600 years. Most medical doctors will not recommend herbs for treatment. One may ask why? Because they do not have many studies on herbal medicine. They are traditionally trained to prescribe medicine. Based on your symptoms they would treat one part of your illness. Herbs do the exact opposite of treating only one system. They actually treat the entire body. Medical

☥

 professionals do not try to cure you of any disease or sickness. Because overall if they keep you brainwashed the doctors and pharmaceutical companies make more money. If they cured anyone they would be out of business.

Let us go back to our ancient healing. The way our ancestors healed people was from herbal plants and spiritual practices. Herbal medicine has been around for millions of years. We need to give our bodies the right nourishment to stay healthy. The only way to do that is to change our lifestyle and heal our bodies the ancient ways and that is with herbs.

"Man is not the flesh nor the body. Man is and will always be the spirit."
~Kemetic Provebs~

☥

The ANKH

The "Ankh" known as the key of life, is the ancient Egypt (Kemet) hieroglyphic character that read "eternal life." Kemetic gods are often seen with this ankh symbol. The oval shape is considered "The womb of life" or "The universe of the woman." The sides of the ankh represent the fallopian tubes. The long piece is the vaginal canal. The ankh is the Kemetic symbol of womb, meaning "eternal life."

The infinite essence of the life that flows in eternal circle.

Goddess Maat

Ancient Kemetic (Egyptian) Goddess Maat represents cosmic order, justice, balance and truth. She is often depicted holding an ankh in her hand, a pair of wings attached to her arms, and a feather in her hair. She is the daughter of the sun god Ra/Raat. The Kemetic culture was centered around order and everything had its natural place in this life. Maat kept everything in motion to maintain harmony and balance on earth. Goddess Maat weighed the heart of the deceased, balanced by her white feather. If the person lived according to Maat the scale would be balanced and the spirit was allowed to go to the afterlife. If the person's heart was overloaded with evil doings and lived against Maat, their heart was devoured by a demon and death was the end result. Keeping our hearts as light as a feather is done by living according to the divine laws of Maat.

☥

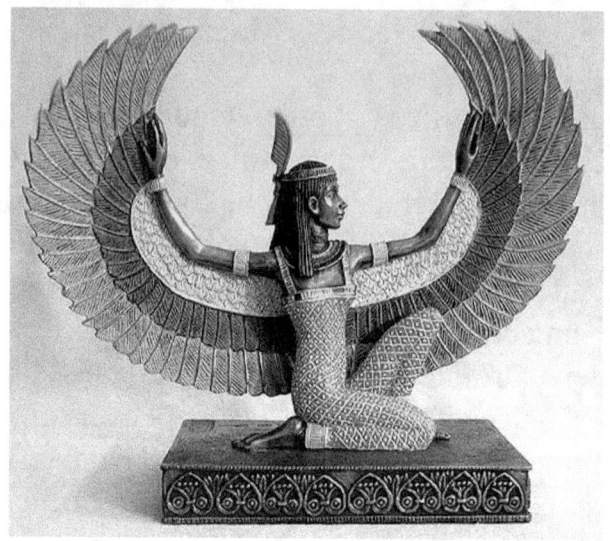

42 Laws of Maat

Thousands of years ago our ancient ancestors lived by these universal laws of Maat, which governed their entire lives daily. Everyone had order, balance, harmony, justice, and truth. There was no need for government, police officers, prisons, or state officials. Everyone was in tuned with nature and obeyed these divine laws.

1. I WILL NOT DO WRONG
2. I WILL NOT STEAL
3. I WILL NOT ACT WITH VIOLENCE

4. I WILL NOT KILL
5. I WILL NOT BE UNJUST
6. I WILL NOT CAUSE PAIN
7. I WILL NOT WASTE FOOD
8. I WILL NOT LIE
9. I WILL NOT DISRESPECT HOLY PLACES
10. I WILL NOT SPEAK EVIL
11. I WILL NOT ABUSE MY SEXUALITY
12. I WILL NOT CAUSE THE SHEDDING OF TEARS
13. I WILL NOT DO SOMETHING I SHALL REGREAT
14. I WILL NOT BE AN AGGRESSOR
15. I WILL NOT BE DECEITFUL
16. I WILL NOT LAY WASTE ON THE LAND
17. I WILL NOT BEAR FALSE WITNESS
18. I WILL NOT SET MY MOUTH IN MOTION (AGAINST ANY PERSON)

☥

19. I WILL NOT BE WRATHFUL AND ANGRY EXCEPT FOR A JUST CAUSE
20. I WILL NOT HAVE SEXUAL RELATIONS WITH A MAN'S WIFE
21. I WILL NOT HAVE SEXUAL RELATIONS WITH A WOMAN'S HUSBAND
22. I WILL NOT POLLUTE MYSELF
23. I WILL NOT CAUSE TERROR
24. I WILL NOT POLLUTE THE EARTH
25. I WILL NOT SPEAK IN ANGER
26. I WILL NOT TURN FROM WORDS OF RIGHT AND TRUTH
27. I WILL NOT UTTER CURSES
28. I WILL NOT INITIATE A FIGHT
29. I WILL NOT BE EXCITABLE OR PROVOKE AN ARGUMENT
30. I WILL NOT BE PREJUDICED
31. I WILL NOT BE AN EAVESDROPPER
32. I WILL NOT SPEAK OVERMUCH
33. I WILL NOT COMMIT TREASON AGAINST MY ANCESTORS

34. I WILL NOT WASTE WATER
35. I WILL NOT DO EVIL
36. I WILL NOT BE ARROGANT
37. I WILL NOT CURSE THE MOST HIGH
38. I WILL NOT COMMIT FRAUD
39. I WILL NOT DEFRAUD TEMPLE OFFERINGS
40. I WILL NOT LOOT THE DEAD
41. I WILL NOT MISTREAT CHILDREN
42. I WILL NOT MISTREAT ANIMALS

☥

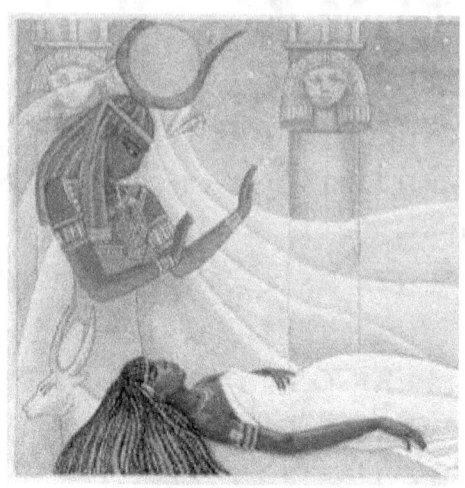

Kemetic Reiki

Kemetic reiki is an ancient healing system utilized by our beloved ancestors throughout Africa and ancient Kemet/Egypt. This healing technique uses universal energy to promote balance and healing for the mind, body, and spirit. You can see from the hieroglyphics left on the pyramid walls in ancient Kemet/Egypt that our ancestors utilized their hands to give and receive energy.

The ancient ones knew how to channel that energy. They had an inner-standing of the energy centers in each one of our hands, particularly the palms. An example is a priest or priestess praying over someone, laying his or her hands over the person, and provoking healing from the Creator. Another example would be massaging your temples, the sides of your head, praying for relief of a headache. Kemetic reiki is used to balance the chakras, clear the aura, and promote healing throughout the entire body. You can choose Kemetic reiki as another way to holistically heal yourself and others. Find a practitioner in your area and schedule your appointment today.

☥

Connecting with your Ancestors

Who is an ancestor? Anyone who has made their transition or one that is descended. We all have come from our ancestors. An ancestor can come from our immediate blood lineage, or from a spiritual elevated lineage. In Traditional African culture we honor our beloved ancestors who came before us. By honoring our ancestors, we make direct connection with their spirits. Some of the many ways we honor and connect with them are the following: Pouring Libation, Ancestry Altars, and Celebrations.

Pouring libation is a great way to show honor and remembrance. A libation is more than just a prayer. It is considered an ancient ritual which involves the pouring of a liquid in offering to a god, spiritual guide, or ancestor. You may utilize any liquid you may choose but, preferably water would be the best choice because of its purity and the fact that it is a natural element. Water has a powerful energetic vibration which lives inside and outside our bodies.

When pouring your libation, make sure you are pure in heart, and have clear intentions when pouring. The first step in connecting with your ancestors is pouring the liquid, so make sure you are fully aware that you are awaking their spirits and they can hear you when doing so. We always start off by thanking our creators (known by many names), our spiritual guides, elements (air, water, fire and earth), four corners (north, east, south and west), and so on. Then we may speak the names of our ancestors. Usually, the libation is acknowledgment and thanks for their divine spirits. We should all know that our beloved ancestors are in the spiritual realm nearby to help us when we may need them. So, not only do we honor them but we continue to ask them for guidance and help along our journey. You may ask for protection, healing, clarity, wisdom, knowledge and so on. Ase' is said at the end, which means "and so it is/let it be."

☥

As a reminder, once you make that connection they do not go away. They are actually closer than before. To make a deeper connection with particular ancestors, say the prayer with conviction and let it be known. You may also have a picture or something symbolic representing the ones you are connecting with. There are many ways when pouring the libation you can pour it on the ground, into a plant, into a natural element such a glass, or you can pour it directly on the floor symbolizing the ground. There are so many ways; these are just a few. Do not be afraid speak from the heart and make the connection.

Your ancestors will speak to you in many different ways; you have to be open to see. Build that relationship and trust. Speak to them regularly by acknowledging their presence. You shall see the difference they can make in your life. We are one with those who came before us. Pouring libation is an African tradition and should be kept in preserving our true culture. ASHE, AMEN RA MAAT

Know Your Life Purpose

Do you know your divine purpose in this lifetime? Each one of us came here in this physical realm to serve a purpose. Are you unsure of what you are supposed to do? Are you content with who you are? Many people live their life with uncertainty of their life purpose, which causes them to live unhappily. Knowing your life path numerology number could clarify your divine purpose.

Easy Steps To Numerology: An Example
1) **Date of Birth**
2) **Add Numbers in Birth Date**
3) **1983**

    +   7

    5
    _____

    1995
4) **Total: 1995**
5) **19**

    + 95
    _____

    114
6) **Total: 114**

☥

7) 11
    + 4
    _____
    15

8) **Total: 15**
9) **Split number in half and add up**
   1 + 5= 6
10)   **Life Path Number is 6**

Now, that you have your numerology life number. Google search your life path number (whatever your number maybe).

Example: Life Path Number 6

People born with a life path number 6 are most incredible nurturers. Home bodied, family oriented, loving, warm, understanding, compassionate, responsible and reliable. Always trying to please others. They make excellent caretakers and providers. They enjoy giving service to others.

Knowing your life purpose makes things a lot easier and you can begin to live your life accordingly. Do not be afraid to **<u>Know Thyself</u>**. Live your life with peace, love, harmony and most of all with MAAT. Stay content in the knowing you are a unique, beautiful, spiritual being. Live a holistic lifestyle and connect with your mind, body and spirit.

☥

"Do MAAT, that your years upon the earth may be long."

~Kemetic Proverbs~

ALSO BY ELAINE DESTINY-BEY

My Diary: Poetry, Situations, Expressions and Affirmations

Vibrant Hair: African-American, Hair Care, Knowledge and Culture

www.destinynatural.com

☥

ABOUT THE AUTHOR

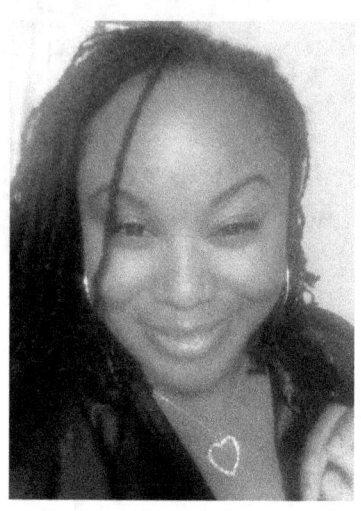

Ms. Elaine Destiny-Bey is the owner of Destiny Natural Wellness & Spiritual Healing, LLC in Las Vegas, Nevada. She is a master teacher in Kemetic Reiki, Herbalist, Author, Healer, Divine Minister, and Educator. Please, feel free to visit her website at: www.destinynatural.com